Thyroid Nᴏᴅᴜ

Questions From Real Patients

By

Shunzhong Shawn Bao, MD

Editor: Barbara Winter

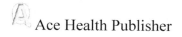

Ace Health Publisher

Publisher's Note/Disclaimer

The information contained herein is not intended to replace the services of a trained health professional or to be a substitute for individual medical advice. You should consult with your healthcare professional regarding to any matter related to your health, and in particular, any matter that may require diagnosis and medical attention.

First Edition 2018

Thyroid Nodules

Questions From Real Patients
Shunzhong Shawn Bao, MD
Barbara Winter, Editor

Published by Ace Health Publisher

Dedication

This book is dedicated to my patients. These are their intelligent questions for which I am grateful. They motivate me to think, continue learning and improving my patient care every day. These days, doctors do not have enough time to address all the questions patients may have. I hope my patients will get some answers here.

I want to thank my nurses, Betty Westbury and Carla Stacks who are providing excellent care to my patients and were the first readers of this book. With their critiques, they have made significant contributions.

This book is also dedicated to my good friend, my editor, Barbara Winter, for her unending kindness and generosity. With her patience and critical editing, she has made this book readable.

Finally, this book is dedicated to my wife who deserves deep, enduring gratitude, and also to my two children who are both in medical school, studying and working very hard. They inspire me to learn and strive for excellence in patient care.

Preface

Because of modern technology such as ultrasound, CT, MRI and PET, we are able to see more abnormal growths in our body which creates more anxiety. Thyroid nodules are an example of abnormal growths that are becoming more prevalent. The language of thyroid nodules is confusing because of terms like "hot nodule," "cold nodule," "warm nodule," "hypoechoic," "RAI," "FNA," "papillary thyroid cancer," etc.

In this book I want to help you understand and learn the language of thyroid nodules by answering real questions from real patients so you will know what your doctors are talking about. I will also discuss what questions to ask your primary care physician, endocrinologist, or surgeon.

This book will not just help you understand thyroid nodules, but it is also a very practical guide for patients addressing very specific questions such as: how to prepare for RAI, should you or should you not be fasting; how to prepare for FNA; what to expect from thyroid surgery; how to take thyroid medications, etc.

I have written this book for patients who have thyroid nodules and also have a family history of either cancerous or noncancerous nodules.

Finally, anyone who is curious and simply wants to learn more about thyroid nodules, will find this book helpful.

Contents

Chapter 3 37

Questions About Thyroid Nuclear Testing............................37

Chapter 7 59

Treatment of Thyroid Nodules: Surgery and Other Modalities 59

Chapter 8 69

Radioactive Iodine Treatment For Thyroid Nodules 69

7

Chapter 1

The basics of thyroid nodule

What is a thyroid?

In English "thyroid gland" is derived from the Latin Glandula Thyreoidea meaning "shield-shaped gland". It is located at the base of your neck.

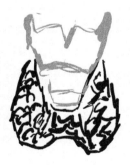

Fig. Illustration of thyroid gland at the base of neck.

The thyroid hormones are T3 and T4. T3 is the active hormone that affects every cell, every tissue, or organ in our body. It is crucial for cells to function properly.

What is a thyroid nodule?

A thyroid nodule is an abnormal growth forming a lump in the thyroid gland. It can be solid, cystic (fluid filled), or complex (partially cystic). It can be on the surface of your thyroid which may be palpable. You or your doctor might feel it. It can form on the inside of your thyroid and not be palpable.

What is a toxic nodule?

If the nodule secretes too much thyroid hormone, we call the nodule toxic. For questions about "hot" nodules and "cold" nodules see chapter 3.

What is the normal size of a thyroid?

On a thyroid ultrasound, the normal thyroid is usually less than 20 mm measuring from anterior to posterior, the thickness of the middle of the thyroid is less than 5 mm, and the length from superior to inferior is usually around 40-60 mm. The weight is around 15-30 g.

What is a goiter?

Goiter simply means that the thyroid gland is bigger than normal. Some doctors use the above average measurements to define it. If you have a measurement greater than 20 mm from anterior to posterior, or the thickness of the middle of your thyroid is greater than 5 mm, then you have a goiter. I define goiters by thyroid contour. Normal thyroid has a flat anterior contour. If I see a bulging anterior contour, then even if the measurement from anterior to posterior is less than 20 mm, I still consider it a goiter. It can be caused by thyroid nodules, general growth, or Hashimoto's thyroiditis. If the goiter is caused by a nodule or nodules, we call it a nodular goiter.

What causes thyroid nodules?

We are not certain about the causes, but they are clearly related to the following:

1) Iodine deficiency. Studies show that populations with iodine deficiencies have much higher incidences of thyroid nodules.

2) Radiation also has been linked to more nodules and more thyroid cancers.

3) Family history. Thyroid nodules and thyroid cancer also tend to occur in family clusters.

4) Acromegaly. Acromegaly is caused by too much growth hormone produced by the pituitary gland or elsewhere.

5) Smoking. If you are a smoker and have iodine deficiency, your risk for thyroid nodules and goiters is much higher.

6) Environment pollution. Some endocrine disruption chemicals (pollutants) have been identified to cause nodules and abnormal endocrine function. Perchlorate, thiocyanate, and nitrate are all competitive inhibitors of the sodium/iodine symporter (the way iodine gets into thyroid cells). Many compounds, including but not limited to: polychlorinated biphenyls (PCBs), polybrominated diphenylethers (PBDEs), bisphenol-A (BPA) and triclosan, may have direct action on the

thyroid hormone receptor and may cause nodules and goiters.

7) Diabetes. There are also reports that the nodules are more common in patients with diabetes.

8) Female hormones. Thyroid nodules are much more common in females and increase with aging.

How much iodine intake is recommended?

Age	Male	Female	Pregnancy	Lactation
Birth to 6 months	110 mcg*	110 mcg*		
7–12 months	130 mcg*	130 mcg*		
1–3 years	90 mcg	90 mcg		
4–8 years	90 mcg	90 mcg		
9–13 years	120 mcg	120 mcg		
14–18 years	150 mcg	150 mcg	220 mcg	290 mcg
19+ years	150 mcg	150 mcg	220 mcg	290 mcg

* Adequate Intake (AI)

The World Health Organization (WHO), United Nations Children's Fund (UNICEF), and the International Council for the Control of Iodine

Deficiency Disorders (ICCIDD) recommend a slightly higher iodine intake for pregnant women of 250 mcg per day.

What food has a high amount of iodine?

The following food list has high iodine content. If you are recommended to have low iodine food (diet), you should avoid this list.

Food	Approximate Micrograms (mcg) per serving	Percent DV*
Seaweed, whole or sheet, 1 g	16 to 2,984	11% to 1,989%
Cod, baked, 3 ounces	99	66%
Yogurt, plain, low-fat, 1 cup	75	50%
Iodized salt, 1.5 g (approx. 1/4 teaspoon)	71	47%
Milk, reduced fat, 1 cup	56	37%
Fish sticks, 3 ounces	54	36%
Bread, white, enriched, 2 slices	45	30%
Fruit cocktail in heavy syrup, canned, 1/2 cup	42	28%
Shrimp, 3 ounces	35	23%
Ice cream, chocolate, 1/2 cup	30	20%
Macaroni, enriched, boiled, 1 cup	27	18%
Egg, 1 large	24	16%
Tuna, canned in oil, drained, 3 ounces	17	11%

*DV = Daily Value. DVs were developed by the U.S. Food and Drug Administration (FDA) to help consumers compare the nutrient contents of products within the context of a total diet. The DV for iodine is 150 mcg for adults and children aged 4 and older. However, the FDA does not require food labels to list iodine content unless a food has been fortified with this nutrient. Foods providing 20% or more of the DV are considered to be high sources of a nutrient.

Do Americans have iodine deficiency?

Prior to the 1920s, endemic iodine deficiency was prevalent in USA mainly in the Great Lakes, Appalachians, and Northwestern regions. In these geographic areas known as the "goiter belt", 26–70% of children had a clinically apparent goiter. The first iodized salt became available on grocery shelves in Michigan on May 1, 1924. The International Council for the Control of Iodine Deficiency Disorders (ICCIDD) Global Network estimates that the proportion of U.S. households with access to iodized salt now exceeds 90%. The actual household usage of iodized salt is not clear.

More recent National Health and Nutrition Examination Survey (NHANES) measurements indicate that urinary iodine levels have stabilized in the general U.S. population. During 2007–2008, NHANES participants aged 6 years and older had an iodine sufficiency rate of 92%. Among women of reproductive age, the sufficiency rate was 85.4%.

56.9% of pregnant women surveyed during 2005–2008 had iodine insufficiency. That iodine insufficiency rate is worrisome.

How much iodine is in U.S. iodine fortified salt?

Now in the U.S. iodine fortified salt has around 67-71 mcg of iodine per 1.5 g of salt (1/4 teaspoon). If you consume 1.5 g of salt daily, you will have half of the recommended iodine intake if you are a non-pregnant adult.

How much iodine is in sea salt?

Sea salt only has a trace amount of iodine. However you can now find iodine fortified sea salt on the market.

I am taking a multivitamin daily. Can I have iodine deficiency?

Not all multivitamins contain iodine. You will need to look at the contents.

How do I know if I have iodine deficiency?

Since 1920 in the U.S., 90% of the population has access to iodized salt and other sources of iodine such as dairy products, seafood, and grains. The Total Diet Study by the U.S. Food and Drug Administration (FDA) in 2003–2004 reported that the important sources of dietary iodine were dairy and grain products. In the U.S., farmers use iodophor to cleanse the milk cans. Iodine is one of several teat dip formulations available in the U.S. dairy industry. Iodine is occasionally introduced in bread dough by the use of iodate as a bread conditioner. Presently, iodine deficiency in the U.S. is uncommon if you consume dairy products. In my clinic, we do not check iodine levels routinely. However, as you can see above, around 8% of the general population, 15% of women at reproductive age, and 43% of pregnant women have iodine deficiencies.

If you want to be sure, have your 24 hour urine checked. However, usually only the iodine concentration in the urine is considered.

Iodine sufficiency is defined as a median urinary iodine concentration of :
--100-299 ug/L for children and nonpregnant adults
--150-249 ug/L for pregnant women.

I usually use the cutoff point of 150 ug/L for nonpregnant adults, and 200 ug/L for pregnant women.

Will my nodule go away if I start to use iodized salt?

Usually your nodule will not go away. However, if you have an iodine deficiency and your nodules are very small, they might not grow to a clinically significant level. Your goiter will shrink.

Can I have too much iodine?

Yes. When it is too high, it can cause thyroiditis, overactive thyroid, or your thyroid can be suppressed.

You will not have too much if you just drink milk or eat some food with high iodine.

Some over the counter supplements can cause too much iodine.

Some medications like Amiodarone can cause too much iodine.

Is there any food that might cause nodules or goiters?

Consumption of foods that contain goitrogens (substances that interfere with the uptake of iodine in the thyroid) can exacerbate iodine deficiency and then lead to nodule formation and goiters. Foods high in goitrogens include soy and cassava, cabbage, broccoli, cauliflower, and other cruciferous vegetables. Deficiencies of iron and/or vitamin A may also be goitrogenic (capable of causing goiters). These issues are of concern primarily for people living in areas prone to iodine deficiency.

How common are thyroid nodules?

They are very common. If you were to use an ultrasound to exam the general population, 50-70% of people would be found to have thyroid nodules. In reality, only 5-7% are found by patients or physicians. Nodules also increase with age. Most nodules are found by different imaging like CT or MRI of the neck for other reasons, carotid duplex scanning, and PET scans for cancer.

Why are thyroid nodules more common in women?

It is reported that thyroid nodules are four times more common in women than men and their frequency increases with age. It is suspected that this might be related to female hormones like estrogen and progesterone since the thyroid nodules increase in women with more pregnancies.

Why should I care about a thyroid nodule?

With any abnormal growth in endocrine organs, we usually ask three questions:
- Is it secreting excessive hormone(s)?
- Is it affecting any surrounding normal organ or structure?
- Is it cancer?

How do I know I may have an overactive thyroid (hyperthyroidism)?

With a very mild overactive thyroid, you might not feel anything. Laboratory tests must be used to make the diagnosis.

For moderate to severe overactive thyroid (hyperthyroidism), you might have anxiety, palpitations, sweating, tremors (shakiness), anger and irritability, difficulty sleeping, and weight loss. 10% of overactive thyroid patients gain weight. I believe this is due to overeating, since hyperthyroidism increases your appetite significantly.

What are the possible symptoms and signs affecting the surrounding organs?

Most benign nodule(s) do not cause any symptoms. You might have some pressure in the neck especially when you are lying down or turning your head if the nodule is big enough. If the nodules are very large. They might cause difficulty breathing or swallowing.

If you have problems swallowing, choking, aspirating food (coughing), hoarseness, shortness of breath, especially coughing with blood, the risk for malignancy (cancer) is significantly increased.

In what other medical history might my doctor be interested?

Your doctor also is interested in your risks for thyroid cancer such as:

- Family and personal history of thyroid disease.
- Family and personal history of thyroid cancer.
- Family history of medullary thyroid cancer (MTC).
- Personal history of head and neck irradiation.
- Personal history of acromegaly.
- Family or personal history of multiple endocrine neoplasia type II.
- Family or personal history of Cowden syndrome (PTEN hamartoma tumor syndrome)
- Family or personal history of Gardner syndrome.
- Family or personal history of adenomatous polyposis.

What is familial medullary thyroid cancer?

It is a more aggressive thyroid cancer. It is derived from a specific cell called a c cell which can secrete calcitonin (a hormone secreted from thyroid to regulate calcium). It can be part of familial medullary thyroid cancer or multiple endocrine neoplasia type II. Luckily, it is rare and comprises only 3% of thyroid cancers.

What is multiple endocrine neoplasia type 2?

Multiple endocrine neoplasia type 2 (MEN2) is subclassified into two distinct syndromes: types 2A (MEN2A) and 2B (MEN2B). Within MEN2A, there are four variants: classical

MEN2A, MEN2A with cutaneous lichen amyloidosis (CLA), MEN2A with Hirschsprung disease (HD), and familial medullary thyroid cancer (FMTC). MEN2B is even rare in comparison to 2A. MEN2B is characterized by medullary thyroid cancer and pheochromocytoma but not hyperparathyroidism. MTC occurs in almost all patients.

What is Cowden syndrome?

Cowden syndrome is caused by gene mutation usually with family history. It is characterized by numerous non-cancerous tumors called hamartomas on the skin or membrane (inside the mouth). Patients with Cowden syndrome have a much higher risk developing thyroid cancer, breast cancer, and gastrointestinal tract cancer.

What is familial adenomatous polyposis?

Familial adenomatous polyposis is an inherited disorder. It usually develops benign colon polyps first and then develops into cancer. It also increases risks for other cancers like adrenal gland and thyroid cancer.

What is Gardner syndrome?

Gardner syndrome is a subset or branch of familial adenomatous polyposis. It also has many tumors in the bone (osteoma) and skin (sebaceous cysts, dermoid cysts, fibroma).

What is the most common symptom of thyroid nodules?

The most common of thyroid symptoms are no symptoms at all. Most nodules are found incidental due to images such as

CT or MRI for the neck or by carotid artery ultrasounds. The nodules found by patients themselves or by physicians are only 5-7%.

Do I need to have a thyroid ultrasound screening for thyroid nodules?

The ultrasound screening for thyroid nodules is not recommended for the general population. However, if you have a family history of thyroid cancer especially in multiple family members, the screening may be reasonable.

If you have a family history of familial adenomatous polyposis, Cowden syndrome, or Gardner syndrome, a thyroid ultrasound for nodule screening may be recommended.

If you have a family history of medullary thyroid cancer or MEN II, then the thyroid ultrasound screening is strongly recommended.

What is the cancer risk for a nodule? Do all nodules have same risk for cancer?

Generally speaking, there is a 5-7% cancer possibility for every single nodule.

Every nodule has a 5-7% risk for thyroid cancer in the adult population. In the pediatric population (<17 years old), the cancer risk is much higher at 26%.

Not all nodules have the same risk. Based on a thyroid ultrasound profile we can decide the cancer risk and then determine if we need to proceed with Fine Needle Aspiration (FNA-see Chapter 5) or other tests.

Chapter 2

Understanding Thyroid Function Tests

How is thyroid function regulated?

Lots of important hormones are regulated by the hypothalamus and pituitary gland. The pituitary gland is a central command for many hormones. It is situated at the base of the brain behind the nose. The hypothalamus secretes a hormone called the thyroid releasing hormone (TRH). It then promotes the pituitary gland to release another hormone called the thyroid stimulating hormone (TSH). TSH then stimulates the thyroid to synthesize and release thyroxine (T4) and triiodothyronine (T3).The levels of T3 and T4 regulate TSH by feedback.

What is TSH?

TSH is a hormone secreted from the pituitary gland. It works like a thermostat. If the T3 and T4 levels are too low, then it turns up the TSH levels. If the T3 and T4 levels are too high, then it shuts down the TSH levels.

TSH regulates T4 and T3 release just like the thermostat regulates your house temperature. TSH is like the thermostat; T4, T3 are like the temperature at your house. If the temperature is too high, your thermostat will shut down; if the temperature is too low, your thermostat will start up. Same thing if your T4 and T3 are too high, TSH will decrease; if T4 and T3 are too low, TSH will increase. Certainly, the assumption is that your thermostat works properly; likewise your pituitary works properly.

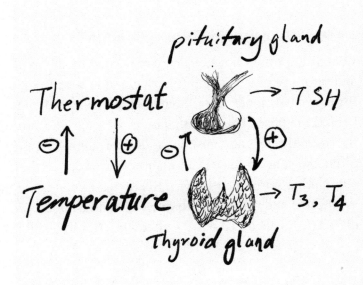

Fig. Illustration of the relationship of the pituitary hormone TSH and T3 and T4 just like a thermostat and the temperature. + indicating stimulating to cause T3 and T4 or temperature to increase; - indicating suppressing (feedback) to cause TSH to decrease or thermostat to shut down, and then T3 and T4, and temperature to decrease.

What is the normal value for TSH?

Different labs might give different normal values. Most labs give a normal value of 0.5-5 mIU/L.

At different ages, the normal value is slightly different. When we age the TSH value tends to increase slightly.

At each stage in pregnancy the TSH levels are different.

What non-thyroid conditions and drugs might affect TSH levels?

Some specialists and professional societies only recommend checking TSH levels which can miss the full picture since TSH can be affected by many conditions and medications.

If you are very sick, your TSH can be low.

Lots of medications also affect TSH values. The most common medications are steroids, dopamine agonists (bromocriptine, cabergoline), somatostatin (a hormone from the pituitary gland or another gland to suppress other hormone secretion), amphetamine, metformin (diabetes medication), amiodarone (heart medication), rexinoids, and opioids.

Is it true that taking too high a dose of biotin can affect TSH measurement?

Yes, biotin might affect the laboratory measurement but not its function.

How are T3 and T4 measured?

Under normal conditions, our thyroid secretes 80% T4 and 20% T3. Most circulating T3 are converted from T4 to T3 at peripheral tissues like liver, kidney. For T4, in blood, 99.98% are bound to proteins (thyroxine-binding globulin, transthyretin and albumin), while 99.80% of T3 is bound to proteins.

It is much easier and much accurate to measure the total hormone (protein bound+free). However, many conditions and medications can affect binding protein levels and then falsely affect the total hormone level. Therefore I do not order the test very often. Unfortunately, the measurement for free hormones are not very accurate either.

What medications increase the total hormones but do not affect thyroid's function?

- Estrogens
- Birth control pills
- Tamoxifen(for breast cancer)
- Mitotane
- Heroin
- 5-fluorouracil (5-FU, cancer medication)
- Methadone(addiction medication)

If you are told you have high thyroid hormone levels, you need to let your doctor know you are on these medications.

What medications decrease the total hormones but do not affect its function?

Some medications can reduce the thyroid binding proteins and then the total hormone levels.

- Androgens (testosterone and similar hormones)
- Glucocorticoids (like prednisone)
- Lithium (can cause thyroid dysfunction)
- Phenytoin
- Propranolol (also inhibit the conversion from T4 to T3)
- Niacin (nicotinic acid)

What conditions increase thyroid hormone binding proteins and then increase the total hormones with normal thyroid function?

The following conditions might increase thyroid binding protein and then increase the total hormone measurement:

- Pregnancy
- Acute /chronic liver disease (can go both ways)
- Adrenal insufficiency
- AIDS
- Familial dysalbuminemic hyperthyroxinemia is a type of hyperthyroxinemia associated with mutations in the human serum albumin gene.
- Familial hyperthyroxinemia due to increased thyroxine binding protein.

What conditions decrease thyroid binding proteins and then reduce the total thyroid hormones with normal thyroid function?

The following conditions might reduce the thyroid binding proteins and cause the measurement of total hormones to be decreased:

- Critical illness (very sick)
- Sepsis (blood infection)
- Nephrotic syndrome (lots of protein lost from kidney)
- Diabetic ketoacidosis (please read my diabetes book)
- Acute and chronic liver diseases (can go both ways)
- Chronic alcoholism
- Severe cirrhosis
- Severe malnutrition
- Acromegaly (enlarged body parts caused by a brain tumor)
- Cushing's syndrome or Cushing's disease (caused by an over abundance steroids in the body)
- Familial thyroxine binding protein deficiency (gene mutation)

How do we measure Free T4 and Free T3?

The free unbound hormones are active, making more sense to measure the free hormones. However, the measurement is not so accurate due to the very low level of the free hormones. Again, only 0.02% of T4 are free hormone and 0.2% of T3 are free hormone.

There are two ways to measure Free T4 and Free T3:
- Estimation of Free T4 and Free T3 testing.

- Use two assays to check both total T3, T4, and binding proteins and then calculate the index.
- Use automated immunoassay-most commonly clinically used.
- Direct measurement. It is very technically demanding and not routinely performed. In very special rare situations, I might order it.

What medication can affect automated immunoassay? I have an abnormal thyroid function test but my function is normal.

Here are the common medications:
- Artificially increase Free T4
  - Amiodarone (can truly increase T4 synthesis)
  - Salicylate (greater than 2g/day)
  - NSAIDS(nonsteroidal anti-inflammatory drugs)
  - Biotin
  - Heparin use
- Artificially decrease Free T4
  - Seizure medication: Phenytoin(dilantin)
  - Seizure medication: carbamazepine

What is TPO?

TPO represents thyroperoxidase, but when we are talking about it most people are talking about the antibody of TPO. It is reported as a titer like 1: 120. When it is high, it usually means you have autoimmune thyroid disease.

Does TPO increase the risk of thyroid cancer?

It is reported that patients with autoimmune disease have higher risks for thyroid cancer. However, it is not concrete. Up until now, no professional societies suggest that you have to screen for thyroid cancer if you have an autoimmune thyroid disease like Hashimoto's thyroiditis.

There is no concrete data suggesting that thyroid nodules in a patient with increased TPO antibody have a higher risk for cancer.

Why is my TPO up and down?

The unstable nature of autoimmune disease is the cause of TPO increasing or decreasing, but also remember the testing is not often accurate. The lab sometimes changes different assays which also makes patients and doctors confused.

Therefore, please do not be too alarmed about TPO variations. I do not recommend checking them repeatedly.

Is there any treatment for increased TPO?

There is no concrete treatment. Some report that selenium might help it. I recommend patients to take 100 mcg of selenium (or selenomethionine 200 mcg) daily. In some patients TPO decreases with the selenium supplement.

Can I take too much selenium?

Yes, you can have too much. We call it selenosis. We can check your blood level. If your blood level of over 100 mcg/dl, you have too much selenium. If you have too much selenium in your blood, you might develop nail problem, hair loss, skin rash, fatigue and increased irritability. Some also reported garlic smelled breath.

If more severe and long term, some cases of skin cancer, liver and kidney damage are reported. I also saw reports that the overdose of selenium is linked to developing of diabetes.

What food do you recommend to increase my selenium level?

Healthy food like nuts and vegetables like spinach has good level of selenium.

What is thyroglobulin? Do I have higher thyroid cancer risks if my value is high?

Thyroglobulin is secreted from normal thyroid follicular cells. It correlates to thyroid volume. The bigger the thyroid tissue, the higher the thyroglobulin. If the thyroid is inflamed, the value also increases.

The high values do not increase the risk for thyroid cancer. Before surgery, I usually do not measure it.

When do you measure thyroglobulin?

If you are confirmed to having thyroid cancer (papillary or follicular) after surgery and/or radioiodine ablation, we measure it to monitor thyroid cancer recurrence.

What is calcitonin?

Calcitonin is a hormone secreted by parafollicular cells (c cells) in response to increased calcium. The thyroid cancer derived from c cells is called medullary thyroid cancer. It is found in 3-5% of all thyroid cancers.

Should I have calcitonin checked in evaluating my thyroid nodule?

I do not recommend checking calcitonin routinely in evaluating thyroid nodules unless you have been suspected to have medullary thyroid cancer by biopsy, by family or personal history of MEN2, familial medullary thyroid cancer, or pheochromocytoma.

I also check calcitonin on patients who have a biopsy showing follicular lesions including Hurthle cell lesion.

Do I need to be fasting before a thyroid function test?

No, you do not need to be fasting for thyroid function test.

Should I take my thyroid supplement on the day of testing?

Your total and free T4 and T3 might increase slightly for the first 4 hours after you take your medication. Your TSH will not be changed.

I recommend my patients do whatever they usually do on the day of testing. No fasting and taking their medication as usual is recommended.

Some patients like to be fasting because they are accustomed. It is okay with me.

Chapter 3

Questions About Thyroid Nuclear Testing

Why are we doing thyroid scintigraphy (nuclear testing-usually an iodine uptake and scan)?

For many years, it was found that "hot" nodules are rarely malignant. This is why sometimes, we want to find out if your nodule is "hot" or "cold".

What is a "hot" nodule? What is a "cold" nodule? What is a "warm" nodule?

A "hot" nodule means the activity in the nodule is higher than the surrounding thyroid tissue. This means the nodule is producing too much thyroid hormones. "Cold" nodule means the activity in the nodule is low. This means the nodule is not producing or under-producing thyroid hormones. "Warm" nodule means the activity is the same as surrounding tissue.

Are all "cold" nodules malignant?

The answer is a big NO. In reality, 80% of nodules are "warm" or "cold". Only 10% of these nodules are malignant. The majority of "cold" nodules, almost 90% are benign.

What should I do if I have a "cold" nodule?

If you have not had an ultrasound, you will need one since cystic nodules are "cold" but predominantly benign.
For most patients, you might need fine needle aspiration (FNA discussed in detail in Chapter 5).

Are all "hot" nodules benign?

The answer is no, but the rate is much lower. 1% of "hot" nodules are estimated to be malignant.

When do doctors order a thyroid iodine uptake and scan test?

When a thyroid nodule is found, the iodine uptake and scan are not the first-line nor last-line test. Most of the time, we do not need this test.

I only order it when the TSH is low. When TSH is low, it means the thyroid function is high (over active thyroid). As we stated before, many reasons can cause low TSH. Thyroid iodine uptake and scan can help us determine to differentiate the causes.

What is the best isotope for thyroid scintigraphy?

I-123 is the most common isotope used for thyroid scintigraphy. The dose usually given is 200-400 uCi.

Does the radioactive iodine uptake and scan hurt my thyroid?

The dose used for iodine uptake and scan is very small. The effect on the thyroid is minimal and we only do it if you have an overactive thyroid.

However, we do want to make sure you are not pregnant if you are a female at reproductive age.

What precautions do I need to take after a radioactive iodine uptake and scan?

The dose is so small. You really do not need to take any precautions, but I recommend washing your hands well after using bathroom and do not handle other people's food and drinks for two days. Do not stay close to a pregnant woman or an infant for two or three days. Do not have sex for three to four days.

Do I need to stay away from certain foods before the test?

One week before the test, I recommend staying off:
- iodine vitamin supplements/iodized salt,
- seaweed (kelp, etc), agar containing food, seafood
- dairy products

Do I need to stay away from certain medications before the test?

You need to stop:
- Antithyroid medication for one week
- Levothyroxine three to four weeks

- Triiodothyronine (Cytomel, T3) one to two weeks
- Topical iodine two to three weeks
- Amiodarone up to six months
- Avoid iodine contrast mediums for CT scans for six weeks to six months prior. Currently, with the commonly used contrast you usually need to wait six weeks.

Do I need to be fasting before the test?

You are recommended to fast 8 hours before the test. However, two hours after you take the pill you are allowed to eat.

How is the test done?

- The test is usually performed at a nuclear department in a hospital.
- After taking the pill, you will be asked to be back in four hours and then the next day for the thyroid scan.
- The scan usually only takes four to five minutes.

Can I have an MRI scan for my thyroid nodule?

There are reports of having MRI scans for indeterminate nodules. However, no professional society supports this practice yet. The insurance companies might not pay for this procedure.

If I have an MRI scan for other reasons and I was found to have a thyroid nodule. What should I do?

You need to have your thyroid function checked, a thyroid ultrasound and followed up with an FNA if needed.

Can I have a PET scan for my thyroid nodule?

There are reports that a PET scan has some value in diagnosing the indeterminate nodules. Again, no professional society recommends PET scans for thyroid nodule evaluation.

However, if you had thyroid cancer and were treated but have a persistent disease process, a PET scan can be considered for further evaluation.

When should I have a thyroid CT scan or MRI?

If your nodule is so big that your doctor cannot get the full picture of your thyroid, a CT or MRI might be ordered to look at the thyroid size and the extension in relationship to surrounding structures, especially with retrosternal extension(extension in the chest).

If a CT is ordered, usually non-contrast is recommended. High iodine in the contrast might cause hyperthyroidism.

What should I do if I was found to have a thyroid nodule on a PET scan performed for other reasons?

If you did not have a thyroid ultrasound before, you will have one to further evaluate the nodule and most likely will also an Fine Needle Aspiration (FNA).

Chapter 4

Thyroid ultrasound

What does a normal thyroid ultrasound look like?

The normal thyroid is very smooth and consistency is very good. It looks whiter than muscle. Here is my own thyroid ultrasound.

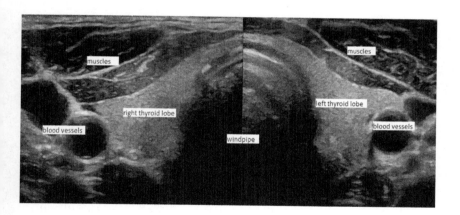

Figure. Normal thyroid ultrasound.

Shunzhong Shawn Bao, MD

My primary care doctor has already completed a thyroid ultrasound. Why does my endocrinologist want to repeat the exam?

The quality of a thyroid ultrasound depends on many factors, such as the training of the operator (reader), patient positioning, patient habitus(or size), quality of the machine, and appropriate machine parameters.

An endocrinologist is trained for administering thyroid ultrasounds and know what to look for. He or she can use different techniques to examine the thyroid in real time, not just by reading the report.

The thyroid ultrasound report you get from your PCP has already has a long journey. You PCP ordered the exam. The technician did the exam and took some pictures. The radiologist reviewed the order and the pictures. He then dictated and the transcriber wrote up the report and hopefully the radiologist reviewed the report and everybody in the chain communicated the information correctly.

I saw a patient for a neck lump. I got a ultrasound report which did not talk about the lump at all since the technician only did thyroid ultrasound and the lump is not in the thyroid.

What does my endocrinologist look for in terms of a thyroid nodule exam on ultrasound?

In dealing with thyroid nodules endocrinologists like to profile nodules with certain patterns tend to be benign while other patterns tend to be associated with a very high risk for malignancy.

44

Following are the features a trained endocrinologist looks for:
- Location: Where is the nodule located?
- Composition: The cystic and spongiform compositions are believed to be benign signs. The nodule can be:
  - cystic
  - spongiform
  - predominantly cystic
  - predominantly solid
  - solid
- Echogenicity (the whiteness and darkness on ultrasound): The malignant chance is much higher if darker-hypoechoic or very hypoechoic.
  - hyperechoic (whiter on the picture than surrounding thyroid tissue)
  - isoechoic (same as the surrounding thyroid tissue)
  - hypoechoic (darker than the surrounding thyroid tissue)
  - very hypoechoic (even darker than neck muscle on ultrasound)
- Shape of the nodule:. Taller than wide has an increased risk for malignancy
- Size: If the size increases, the risk for malignancy also increases.
- Margin (edge):A smooth margin has higher chances for being benign.
  - Smooth, spherical or elliptical nodules with well-defined edges are favorable.
  - Irregular, with speculated, jagged, or sharp angles with protrusions into the surrounding thyroid tissue is not favorable.

- ○ Lobulated, rounded large protrusions into the surrounding tissue is not favorable.
  - ○ Ill-defined, unable to clearly define the margin, is not favorable.
  - ○ Halos: a dark border at the periphery of the nodule, if a complete circle, is favorable.
  - ○ Extrathyroidal extension where the nodule has broken through the thyroid capsule is very high risk, most unfavorable.
- Calcification.
  - ○ punctate (microcalcification)-not favorable
  - ○ macrocalcification/coarse calcification-neutral
  - ○ peripheral calcification/broken edge calcification. If complete it is favorable; if broken it is not favorable

If a nodule has multiple unfavorable features, then the risk for malignancy is drastically increased.

How do I prepare for a thyroid ultrasound exam?

You do not really need any preparation. I recommend you wear a low cut shirt that makes the lower neck and thyroid area easily accessed.

Is there any harm to me?

We have not identified any harm or side effects for a thyroid ultrasound.

What is involved in a thyroid ultrasound exam?

We require you to lie flat and, if possible, to put a pillow under your shoulders to extend your neck.

What ultrasound patterns show high suspicion(70-90% risk)?

When I see the following ultrasound features, I know the nodule has a very high risk for cancer. Basically any combination of two or more unfavorable features. Certainly, the more unfavorable feature, the higher the risk.

- Hypoechoic (darker) with unfavorable margin including irregular margin, undefined margin, lobulated margin, broken "eggshell" calcification with extension to outside of "eggshell", or extrathyroid extension
- Hypoechoic (darker) with microcalcification
- Hypoechoic (darker) with taller than wide
- Any nodule with neck suspicious lymph node
- I consider any nodule with unfavorable margin features as very high risk. However, ATA (American Thyroid Association) did not put this in their high suspicious group

What are the intermediate risk ultrasound features?

Any nodule with hypoechoic solid nodule but without other high risk features, especially with regular margins, has a 10-20% risk for thyroid cancer.

What are the low risk ultrasound features?

Any isoechoic or hyperechoic nodule with or without cystic changes (solid greater than 50%), and with regular margins are low risk. The cancer risk is between 5% and 10%. I usually do not proceed with a FNA unless the size is greater than 1.5 cm.

What are the very low risk ultrasound features?

If I see a spongiform nodule or dominantly cystic nodule (the cystic part greater than 50%) without any other high risk features like irregular margin or a suspicious lymph node, I know these nodules have less than 3% risk of malignancy. I usually do not proceed with FNA unless it is greater than 2 cm in size.

What is the benign thyroid ultrasound feature?

Pure cystic nodules are rarely cancerous. The risk is less than 1%. I usually do not do a FNA unless nodule is too big and causing some uncomfortable symptoms.

Chapter 5

Thyroid Nodule Fine Needle Aspiration (FNA)

What is a thyroid nodule fine needle aspiration?

Using a very small needle (usually smaller than 25 gauge) some cells are secured to be examined by a pathologist. We may also use the material for a gene mutation tests done to increase the predictability of benign or malignancy. If a parathyroid adenoma is suspected, we also measure the parathyroid hormone in a FNA washout.

If we have to do a FNA for a lymph nodes in conjunction with thyroid cancer, we will measure the thyroglobulin in the FNA washout.

Why should I have an FNA?

As discussed before, whenever we find something growing in your body, we ask three fundamental questions: is it functional? Is it compromising the function of surrounding cells, tissue or organs? Is it cancer?

49

FNA is the most important procedure to make the diagnosis of cancer before surgery.

After introducing the technique, the malignant rate of thyroid increased from 14% to 50%. This means that more people avoid surgery due to a benign diagnosis from an FNA.

Therefore, a FNA is to make sure the nodule is not malignant and you do not have to have surgery.

Can I continue to take blood thinner?

You should continue to take blood thinner. However, your risk for bleeding is increased and the chance of having a non-diagnostic result is increased.

Is it very painful?

You can expect to have some pain but it is not excruciating. I usually give some lidocaine using a very small needle (30-31 gauge). Lidocaine itself can cause localized burning pain.

Some physicians do not give any anesthetics. I find it better to give some lidocaine.

What can I take for the pain?

You can take some Tylenol or Ibuprofen if you want. Ice packs are very effective and can reduce swelling and bruising.

What do I need to prepare for an FNA?

You do not need to specifically prepare for anything. You will be awake. You can eat and drink water, but be careful not to get too much. Some feel nauseated during the procedure. It is a good idea to empty your bladder just before the procedure.

You will be required to lie flat. I recommend that you wear a low cut shirt or sweater so you do not need to change.

How is the procedure done?

You will need to lie flat on an exam table with a pillow under your shoulders to extend your neck so your thyroid will be better exposed.

Most doctors use alcohol (others includes iodine and chlorhexidine) to disinfectant and sterilize the area.

Then a little ultrasound gel (usually cold) will be put on the base of your neck. I usually inject some 1% lidocaine to help reduce the pain. The lidocaine might cause an uncomfortable burning in the area of injection..

Then a 25 gauge needle will be used to make a few passes into the nodule under ultrasound guidance.

You will be instructed not to swallow, cough, or speak during the procedure.

I had a shooting pain to my ear during the procedure. What was happening?

There are nerves supplying your upper neck and ear that goes through the thyroid area. The needle might hit one of those nerves, but it will not damage your nerve.

What can I expect after the procedure?

You are allowed to drive home immediately. You will not have restrictions for any activity. Singing too loudly might cause some pain. I recommend you not talk too much, and not sing for one or two days.

After the lidocaine wears off, you can expect to have some pain. If you want, you can take some ibuprofen or Tylenol.

Bruises are very common. They might take up to seven days to go away. Using an ice pack after getting home might reduce your pain and bruising.

What complications might an FNA cause?

Before the procedure you are asked to sign a consent to acknowledge the following possible complications. These complications are very rare but they do occur:
- Bleeding (most occur inside the thyroid nodule)
- Infection
- Bruising
- Thyroid swelling, tracheal damage, recurrent laryngeal nerve damage

When should I call my doctor's office or go to ER?

If you have unusual neck or swallowing pain, especially associated with fever, you need to call your doctor. If you have trouble breathing, you need to go to ER. Otherwise you can just take some Tylenol or Ibuprofen for pain. It is recommended to have ice pack for swelling and pain and may also reduce bruising.

Chapter 6

The Possible Results of FNA and Course of Action

What are the possible results?

We use the Bethesda system to report the thyroid FNA results. :

- Non-diagnostic or unsatisfactory
- Benign
- Atypia of undetermined significance (AUS) or follicular lesion of undetermined significance(FLUS)
- Follicular neoplasm or suspicious for follicular neoplasm
- Suspicious for malignancy
- Malignant

I received a call from my doctor's office saying the FNA result is non-diagnostic or unsatisfactory. What does this mean?

In order for a pathologist to decide if the biopsy is benign or not, it is necessary to see at least six groups of thyroid cells of at least ten cells in a group.

There is between a 5-20% chance for a nodule to be found in this category. The exact reason is not clear, but **studies show that the cancer rate in this** category **is actually very low at 1-4%.**

Here are a few reasons I suggest:
- Your nodule might be too small to have a FNA
- Your nodule has a cystic component. The cystic component might be due to the liquidation of living cells. In other words, even the FNA is sampled from the solid part. The cells may already be dead.
- You might be prone to bleeding. Too many blood cells in the needle dilute the thyroid cells.
- You might be taking blood thinner which can cause bleeding.

What is the recommendation for non-diagnostic and unsatisfactory results?

Since the overall risk for cancer is low (around 1-4%), I usually ask my patients to wait for three months and then we will repeat an ultrasound and make a decision:
- If your nodule has grown in even three months, I might recommend to repeat biopsy or go to have surgery soon.
- If your nodule has many unfavorable features (see above), then I definitely recommend to repeat an FNA or surgery.
- If your nodule is solid but seems to be benign, and you are on blood thinner, I might just continue to follow up with thyroid ultrasound every six months to one year.
- If your nodule is cystic or predominantly cystic, I also recommend continuing to monitor with thyroid ultrasounds instead of repeating an FNA.

My nodule is FNA benign. Now what?

When you have a FNA benign result, your chance of having benign nodule is 99%. Here are my recommendations:

- If your nodule is not much bigger and you do not have other symptoms of significant discomfort, I would usually not recommend surgery. This is why we have FNA. We might follow up with a thyroid ultrasound every 1-2 years or longer.
- If your nodule is benign on the FNA report but you have multiple unfavorable features, I might still recommend having surgery or repeat a thyroid FNA in three to six months.
- If a previous FNAwas benign, but your nodule shows very significant growth, then I would recommend repeating FNA.

My FNA reported as atypia of undetermined significance (AUS) or follicular lesion of undetermined significance(FLUS). What does this mean?

20-25% of FNA are reported as AUS or FLUS. There are some abnormal cells but not enough to suspect cancer.

What is my cancer risk if I have atypia of undetermined significance (AUS) or follicular lesion of undetermined significance(FLUS)?

The cancer risk is 5-15%.

What can we do with these undetermined results?

Here are a few scenarios and my recommendations:

- If you have significant risk factors like a very young age (<16), a history of neck radiation, family history of thyroid cancer, or other genetic diseases highly associated with thyroid cancer, I would recommend surgery.
- If you have a nodule with many ultrasound unfavorable features, I would also recommend surgery.
- If you do not have any of the above, I usually recommend repeating FNA and molecular testing in three to six months. Then, based on the molecular testing result, decide what the next step is.

What is molecular testing?

Thyroid cancers like other cancers have gene mutations. The most common tests available include the Afirma Genomic Sequencing Classifier(GSC), ThyGenX, and ThyroSeq. In my clinic, I use the Afirma GSC. These gene tests are not "bullet proof". Even if molecular testing suggests it to be benign, we still recommend long-term follow up.

What does "follicular neoplasm or suspicious for follicular neoplasm" mean?

This is very challenging to a pathologists as well as an endocrinologists. A pathologist has trouble in determining it to be simply hyperplasia, a tumor, or cancer. An endocrinologist does not know if it is a follicular thyroid cancer or benign follicular neoplasm.

What is the cancer risk for follicular neoplasm or suspicious for follicular neoplasm?

The cancer risk is 15-30%.

What do you recommend if an FNA result is follicular neoplasm or suspicious for follicular neoplasm?

Due to the uncertainty of being benign or malignant, I usually refer to surgery especially for patients with any risk factors. Most recently I had a patient's' FNA reported as a follicular neoplasm but surgery revealed as medullary thyroid cancer which is a very aggressive thyroid cancer. Any report as follicular neoplasm or suspicious for follicular neoplasm, I would also check for calcitonin. Calcitonin can be the cancer marker for medullary thyroid cancer.

For patients who are not good candidates for surgery, I wait three months and repeat FNA plus I order molecular testing. I definitely follow up with thyroid ultrasounds.

My FNA reported malignant(cancerous) or suspicious for malignancy. Can I choose not to have surgery?

For patients whose FNA reported the nodule as possibly malignant, or malignant, I routinely order surgery. There is a movement now trying to do less surgery. It is recommended to have partial thyroidectomy if the tumor is small and no metastatic lymph nodes. It may be okay for patients whose other lobe is very clearly normal findings, otherwise, I recommend to have a total thyroidectomy. I have so many patients who had a lobectomy for a thyroid nodules and now return for a second surgery for nodules in the other lobe.

There are some specialists who recommend not having surgery for small cancers. There are some patients who are not suitable for surgery. This is what I do: Before I do a FNA, I usually discuss with my patients about possible results and what we would do. If patients do not want to have surgery, or are not suitable for surgery, I would not even do the FNA.

What is Hurthle cell neoplasms?

Hurthle cell neoplasm is a subtype of follicular neoplasm. Follicular thyroid cancer with Hurthle cells is more aggressive. I recommend surgery. There are patients with medullary thyroid cancer that was misdiagnosed as Hurthle cell neoplasms.

Are there any other findings from FNA?

Others findings are very rare such as medullary thyroid cancer, poorly differentiated thyroid cancer, anaplastic thyroid carcinoma, lymphoma or metastatic cancer.

Chapter 7

Treatment of Thyroid Nodules: Surgery and Other Modalities

Can you repeat your recommended indications for surgery?

I usually refer patients to have surgery for the following situations:

- The nodule or nodules are very large (usually greater than 4 cm), especially causing some pressure symptoms like severe discomfort, choking, affecting swallowing, or simply cosmetic issues.
- FNA suspicious for possible malignant or malignant nodules.
- FNA for follicular neoplasm or suspicious for a follicular neoplasm; especially patients with some risk factors like a history of neck radiation, a family history of thyroid cancer or other associated cancers, and especially for patients who are unable to have follow up or who have an anxiety disorder.
- FNA benign or undetermined but with multiple ultrasound unfavorable features.

What is involved with thyroid surgery?

You usually will be admitted to the hospital on the day of surgery. You will have general anesthesia which means you will have a breathing tube while undergoing surgery.

A small cut (depending on the type of surgery) will be made at the base of your neck along the skin crease to minimize showing the scar.

The surgery itself usually lasts one to two hours.

The surgical procedure involves proximity to large blood vessels, nerves for voice (recurrent laryngeal nerves as well as the external branches of the superior laryngeal nerve), and also parathyroid (governing your calcium balance).

What questions should I ask my surgeon?

We usually refer you to a surgeon we think is very good, but the relationship needs to be personal. At the consultation, you need to ask questions and see if you feel comfortable letting the surgeon do the job.

- How many thyroid surgeries do you perform annually?
    - Some research reports that surgeons who do over 25 cases per year have fewer complications.
- Do you follow current thyroid surgery guideline? If not, why?
    - Guidelines are very important in deciding how to treat, but the surgeon also needs to understand your specific condition.

- Do I really need surgery? What are the alternatives? Advantages and disadvantages?
    - You are referred to have surgery. This does not mean you have to have surgery.
- What are the possible complications?
- What is your rate of complications?
    - Thyroid surgery can have complications. See below. While asking these questions, you might be able to sense how confident are his or her responses .
    - I do not like the answer "I do not know". I believe when doing anything, if you track what you do, you do better. When a surgeon does not know what his or her complication rate is, then he or she might not focus on improving himself or herself.

- If you have worries for a particular complication such as loss of voice, ask for the last time this happened to his or her patient. What was the possible reason?
- Is there anything the surgeon can do to reduce the risk?
- What is his plan? Based on your condition, what kind of surgery is he or she planning to do?
    - Depending on your current diagnosis, is the surgeon planning to remove just the nodule? Lobectomy? Near total thyroidectomy? Complete total thyroidectomy? Need to remove lymph nodes?
- If you worry about the scar, ask to see if you can get a plastic surgeon for the cut and closing. What product does he or she recommend for your healing? Anything else you need to do to reduce the scar formation? If you

tend to form keloid, tell them now to see if they can do anything.

What are the potential complications for thyroid surgery?

Surgery can have complications, but nowadays surgeons are better too. However, the complication rate is absolutely surgeon dependent. I only refer to surgeons who have lots of experiences and I communicate my perspective for the particular patient to them. The following are the complications which might happen:

- Bleeding, especially for patients with bleeding disorders. This can be very dangerous and life threatening.
- Neck swelling-seroma, causing bulging but no significant pressure symptoms.
- Infection is rare and I have not seen one.
- Nerve damage causing hoarseness. If severe enough, it can cause breathing difficulties.
- Numbness and tingling caused by damage to the parathyroid gland which is very important in maintaining blood calcium level. If calcium is very low and not corrected, it can not only cause spasms but it can also cause irregular heartbeats and be life threatening.
- Surgeon will also discuss other complications with you like anesthesia reactions which can cause death. I remember in the news a girl died in removing a tonsil.

What is my down time for surgery?

Thyroid surgery in most centers involves an overnight stay. Most patients told me that they did not need any pain medication at all.

It is a good idea to stay home for one week. I recommend my patients not to talk too much, yell and not to sing for one week or two.

What are my restrictions after surgery?

Until the first follow-up appointment after surgery, you should restrain from:
- Talking too much, yelling, or singing.
- Bending down or doing any strenuous activity.
- Lifting any heavy objects.
- Driving if you do not have full motion of your neck.

What do I need to pay attention to?

You need to pay attention to the following. If any of the following occurs, do not hesitate to call your surgeon.
- If you have fever, or unusual pain, you might have infection.
- If your neck swells, especially with pressure.
- If you have choking, especially with too much pressure and especially difficulty breathing.
- If you have numbness and tingling, you can try taking more calcium. If not relieved, call your doctor.

I have a scratchy voice, does it mean my vocal cord nerve is damaged?

No. As we stated, you have a breathing tube going between your vocal cords and might have a small degree trauma which causes your scratchy voice. It can take up to one week to heal.

Due to the surgical procedure, the edema, swelling and temporarily compromised blood flow might affect nerve or muscle movement. This can cause some difficulty in speaking. This should improve in a few weeks.

This is one of the reasons I recommend not talking too much, yelling, or singing.

How do I know my voice nerve has been damaged?

If you have difficulty breathing while talking and it is very difficult to speak, then most likely your voice nerves have been compromised.

Do not panic. If you panic, it will make your breathing even more difficult. Your surgeon will help you to find the right physician or speech therapist to help you.

Will I have an ugly scar on my neck?

It actually will depend on your own skin's ability to heal. Some patients that tend to have keloids most likely will have trouble. Most patients will not have an ugly scar. The surgeon will make as small an incision as possible along the skin crease to minimize the scar showing.

If this is very important for you, you need to talk to your surgeon about it. Together you can decide if you need a plastic surgeon to assist for the cut and close.

There is a report of an alternative route from the axilla to make the cut. I do not know any surgeon who does that in my area.

Can I do anything to reduce the scar?

Most people heal well. A cut in the neck usually heals nicely.

I have patients who use silicone gel, or hydrogel and apply it to the incision daily for some extended time (3 months or more). I also have patients who use the Mederma Advanced Scar Gel and believe helps.

You should also protect the scar from sunlight for the first three months. I have patients reported that using sun scream is very helpful.

When you talk to your surgeon, you can ask for more suggestions.

Can we reduce the chance of any complications?

- I refer my patients to a surgeon with a good track record. Different surgeons makes different outcomes.
- I will check your vitamin D and calcium level before surgery. I will start vitamin D supplements before sending you to have surgery.
- Closely monitor your calcium after surgery.
- Have an ENT doctor check your vocal cord before surgery if you have concerns for voices.

65

Do I always need calcium tablets after surgery?

No, this depends on the damage to the parathyroid glands. We have at least four of them, two on each side. If you just have a lobectomy (half of your thyroid removed), you do not need extra calcium since we know at least the other two are working.

If you have a total thyroidectomy and the surgeon is not so sure if he or she can identify the parathyroid glands and preserve them. We can check your PTH the second morning. If they are low, then you need calcium, vitamin D or active vitamin D calcitriol depending on your calcium level. However, before surgery, I always check my patient's vitamin D to make sure they have adequate vitamin D.

When can I get pregnant after thyroid surgery?

I recommend getting your thyroid hormone optimized before becoming pregnant. Thyroid hormone is very important for pregnancy. It is not just for getting pregnant and a healthy pregnancy. It is also crucial for fetal brain development.

Make sure to communicate with your endocrinologist before you become pregnant.

Will thyroid surgery affect my sex life?

You can resume sexual activity as soon as you feel like it. Thyroid surgery itself does not affect your sex life long term, but if you do not have your thyroid hormone balanced, then your sex life can be affected. As we discussed before, thyroid hormone affects every cell, every tissue, every organ in our body. Therefore, after thyroid surgery, you need to follow up with your endocrinologist or internist to make sure your thyroid hormone is balanced.

I heard that some centers use alcohol injection to treat thyroid nodules. What do you think?

At some centers, alcohol is being used to treat benign and simple cystic nodules. I have patients who had the treatment and said the procedure caused very significant pain. Also, the post treatment thyroid ultrasound does not look good which might confuse the treating physicians.

However, if you have access to an experienced physician it should be a safe procedure especially if you have other comorbidities which increase your risk for surgery. This can be a good option for you.

Do I have any other non-surgical options for a thyroid nodule?

For a noncancerous nodules, if the patient does not want to have surgery or surgery is not desirable, some centers offer laser ablation, cryoablation, and radiofrequency ablation to remove the benign nodule. In some circumstances, radioactive iodine is recommended.

Chapter 8

Radioactive Iodine Treatment For Thyroid Nodules

What is radioactive iodine?

Iodine comes in different forms. The radioactive iodine we are talking about here is the form which can emit particles and can kill thyroid cells.

When do you recommend radioactive iodine for thyroid nodule treatment?

I recommend radioactive iodine for thyroid nodule treatment with the following conditions:

- If you have a "hot" nodule or nodules.
- If you do not want to have surgery or surgery is not recommended for you and you have a large goiter which produce symptoms like too much pressure, choking, or difficulty breathing.

How long does the radioactive iodine (radioiodine) stay in your body?

Radioiodine stays in your body for only a short time. The radioiodine that does not go to thyroid tissue will be eliminated from your body during the first few days after treatment. It leaves your body primarily through your urine, but very small amounts can be found in your saliva, sweat, semen, and bowel movements.

I am allergic to seafood or allergic to intravenous iodine contrast. Can I still use it?

Yes, you can. You might be allergic to the iodine carriers but not the iodine itself. Therefore, you are not allergic to radioactive iodine which is a simple iodine salt.

Can I use the radioactive iodine to treat a benign nodule?

Yes and no. If your nodule is overactive, then you can use it. Otherwise, you cannot. However, if you have a goiter this brings some problem for you, if you do not want to have surgery or surgery is not recommended due to other comorbidities (making surgery too risky), then radioactive iodine can be used to shrink the whole thyroid gland,

What is involved in radioactive iodine treatment?

The Endocrinologist or nuclear medicine physician will give you a capsule of radioactive iodine and you take it with a glass of water. That is it. Usually you only need to take it one time. A very small percentage of patients will need second treatment.

I have a single toxic nodule. What should I expect after radioactive treatment for thyroid function?

Your overactive thyroid function can be controlled in 50% of cases in three months, and 80-90% of cases in six months.

Some patients have normal thyroid function; some patients develop low thyroid. There is a 6-50% of chance to have low thyroid function at 6 months. The thyroid function needs to be followed long term. The low thyroid (hypothyroidism) continues to increase with years going by. After six months, if your thyroid function is still normal, I recommend checking it every three to six months. 6-10% of patients will need a second treatment.

The risk for developing low thyroid is increased if pretreatment with antithyroid medication like methimazole or propylthiouracil (PTU). The reason is not very clear to me. I think this might be due to the dose was higher due to the calculation for the iodine uptake and scan. Antithyroid medication reduce the iodine uptake.

I have a toxic multinodular goiter. What should I expect after radioactive treatment?

- You might experience slight pain in the neck in the following days up to a few weeks.
- You might experience neck swelling -with it becoming bigger in the following days or weeks, instead of becoming smaller.
- After two years, about 90% of treatment success (thyroid function is under control) can be achieved. Usually the goiter is smaller.
- 28% (different rate with different reports) of patients develop hypothyroidism (low thyroid) at one year after radioactive treatment. Thyroid functions will need to be monitored long term.

Which would you prefer-surgery or radioactive iodine treatment if you have toxic thyroid nodule?

The decision can be hard. I am in my 50s and my heart is healthy. I am not taking any medications right now. If I have a single toxic nodule or a toxic multinodular goiter, I would prefer to have the radioactive iodine treatment. Here are the reasons:

- Radioactive iodine involves no down time if you work by yourself. Otherwise, I recommend one week off from work.
- The risk is much lower. Although, theoretically it increases your chance to have cancer, the dose is very low and the chance is very, very low.
- I can check my thyroid function regularly to follow my thyroid function.
- I have a 50% chance of not having to take thyroid medication.

When would you prefer surgery over the radioactive iodine procedure?

I would recommend surgery over radioactive iodine for the following scenarios:

- You have developed atrial fibrillation and want to get your hyperthyroid under control as soon as possible.
- You have another heart conditions and want to get hyperthyroidism under control as soon as possible, but you can tolerate surgery. If your cardiologist is not ok with the surgery, we can still recommend medication and then radioactive iodine treatment if necessary.
- Your living conditions do not allow you to follow up with your physician frequently.

- You want it fixed quickly
- Your nodule is so big that it affects your breathing or swallowing.
- You might also have thyroid cancer.
- You have pregnant women or small children at home, you might consider surgery.
- You have been or are taking medications like Amiodarone, you might want to consider sugary.

How do I prepare for radioactive iodine treatment?

- If you are taking an anti-thyroid medication like methimazole or propylthiouracil (PTU), you will need to stop taking it at least three days before. I usually ask my patients to stop five to seven days before the treatment. If the thyroid function is suppressed too low, I ask my patients to stop ten days before the treatment.
- Follow a low iodine diet (see chapter 1 for high iodine diet) for 1-2 weeks if not urgent. This includes avoiding:
  - iodized table salt (sea salt is ok if not iodized)
  - cough medicine
  - seafood
  - vitamin supplements that contain iodine
  - dairy products contain some iodine, so you need to cut down on cheese, milk and milk products
  - eggs

You should also cut out any food colored pink with the additive E127 (more commonly used in Europe) such as:

- spam or salami
- tinned strawberries

- glacé cherries
- pink pastries or sweets (look on the labels for E127)

What should I do if I have been taking high iodine medications like Amiodarone?

Amiodarone has a very high level of iodine and can stay in your body up to ten years. I would recommend surgery if possible. However, I might still order an iodine uptake and scan to see if your thyroid can absorb any iodine. If there is some uptake, we still can treat with radioactive iodine although with a slightly higher dose. The failure rate might be higher. We might also be able to increase the thyroid absorption by giving you a recombinant TSH--Thyrogen.

What should I do if I have recently had a CT scan with a contrast agent?

Many agents have high levels of iodine. However, right now most agents can be eliminated from your body in two weeks if you have normal kidney function. Therefore, you can receive radioactive iodine treatment after a two week wait.

How long should I wait if I have used some topical iodine agent?

You need to wait at least two to three weeks.

Should I fast on the day of treatment?

You should fast overnight because doctors believe that iodine can be absorbed faster. However, it is okay if you have not.

What procedure is involved in this treatment?

If you are a woman at reproductive age, you will need a lab test to confirm that you are not pregnant.

Usually you will be instructed to be on low iodine for at least two weeks. On rare occasions, Thyrogen (recombinant TSH) is given for up to three days.

On the day of treatment, you are instructed fast (okay to drink water). After reviewing the safety procedures, a capsule of radioactive iodine is given to you to take by a nuclear medicine doctor or your endocrinologist. You can eat after one to two hours. Again, if you have not been fasting, it is okay.

What are the side effects of the radioactive iodine treatment?

- **Increased of overactive thyroid:** Radioactive iodine destroys your thyroid, thus more thyroid hormones are released.
- **Metallic taste in the mouth:** This can last for a few weeks.
- **Nausea:** This usually subsides one to two days after treatment. It is okay to take some nausea medications if needed.
- **Swollen salivary glands:** This can last for a few weeks. This is caused by iodine absorbed by the salivary glands. Stimulating saliva flow a few days after treatment by sucking a lemon drop, for instance, is an effective remedy.

- **Dry mouth**: This can be a long term annoying side effect. As recommended, drink plenty of water after the treatment and stimulate saliva flow by using lemon drops or lozenges.
- **Hypothyroidism:** As we discussed, up to 50% or more patients treated with radioactive iodine will develop hypothyroidism or low thyroid. The good news is that this is really easy to treat and if properly treated, there are no side effects.
- **Cancer**: This is a theoretic risk. The real risk is not known.

What can you do to minimize the worsening of an overactive thyroid after treatment?

Usually this is short-lived and I do not worry about it. However, if you are elderly and your thyroid hormones are very high (above two to three times normal limits) with cardiovascular disease, I recommend pretreatment using an anti-thyroid medication like methimazole. This medication needs to be stopped at least three days before the radioactive iodine treatment.

You can also restart anti-thyroid medication.

Sometimes, I also use cholesterol medication Cholestyramine.

When do you restart anti-thyroid medication after radioactive iodine treatment?

I usually do not restart anti-thyroid medications after treatment. If your level is too high or you have a very severe cardiovascular disease I'm worried about your thyroid hormone surging after the treatment. I would restart anti-thyroid medication a day after you take your radioactive iodine treatment. The thyroid function needs to be followed closely.

I also use Cholestyramine after treatment waiting one day after the radioactive iodine treatment.

What can you do to minimize the chance of developing hypothyroidism(low thyroid)?

This can be tricky. Some centers are giving a fixed dose, some centers calculate your dose based on your thyroid mass or nodule, but we are sure if we give you less radioactive iodine your chance to be cured (or control your thyroid function, or shrink your thyroid nodule or goiter) will be reduced. Usually the dose for treating a toxic nodule, a toxic multinodular goiter, or goiter ranges from 10-50 mCi.

When can I get pregnant after radioactive iodine treatment?

It will be verified by a lab test that you are not pregnant when you are treated. It is recommended not to get pregnant for at least six months. Ideally, do not get pregnant for 12 months especially if you plan to breast feed.

Do I need to bank my sperm before receiving iodine treatment?

Usually the dose used for a toxic thyroid nodule or a toxic multinodular goiter is relatively small. Although radioactive iodine can cause sperm counts to decrease, the fertility decrease is not clinically significant. It is not recommended for you to bank your sperm. However, if you know your sperm count is low to begin with, it is not a bad idea.

If you have metastatic thyroid cancer and are expected to have multiple rounds of radioactive iodine treatments, then banking your sperm is very reasonable.

When can I impregnate my wife after radioactive iodine treatment?

There is no specific recommendation but this does not mean it is safe, therefore I recommend you wait for three months.

When can I resume sexual activity?

I recommend no sex for two weeks. Condoms are strongly recommended especially for men treated with radioactive iodine.

After treatment can I take public transportation home?

I strongly discourage you from taking public transportation home to minimize your exposure to the public. If you are well enough, I recommend you drive home.

However, if you have to take public transportation home, sit as far away as possible from other people, especially from children or pregnant women.

Is there a time limit for taking public transportation?

Yes, again, I recommend you not take public transportation if possible on the first day. If you do, for the first day limit to two hours, then for the second day limit to three hours, the third day limit to four hours, and the fourth day limit to five hours. Airplane travel is strongly discouraged for a week after treatment.

When can I ride in an airplane and any precautions?

I recommend against air travel the first week, especially the first three days. Sometimes even after a week you still have radioactive iodine in your system and can trigger the alarm system in the airport. If you must travel, you might ask your treating physician to write a letter for you.

Do I need to obtain anything specific for the treatment?

Not really if you can take care of yourself. If you need other people to take care of you, or you have some specific conditions like a stool bags (colostomies) or urine bags, then you need to get good gloves and wipes for your helper. Also obtain bags to store the materials you cannot flush down the toilet.

Shunzhong Shawn Bao, MD

Should I stay at hospital after treatment?

Usually you are released at the same day.

Should I stay in a hotel to minimize contaminating my own house?

A hotel is a public house so I do not recommend going to a hotel for that reason. However, due to your household situation, if you have small children or pregnant women at home and you are not able to stay six feet away (briefly passing by is okay), you might consider staying in a hotel. If you do, please take precautions as at your own home.

If you are treated for toxic nodule or nodules, a three to four day stay at hotel should be enough. If you have thyroid cancer and are treated with radioactive iodine, a week long stay is more appropriate.

How long should I stay at home before going back to work?

If possible, you should stay at home for a week.

At night, how long should I sleep in a separate bedroom or beds at least six feet apart?

- Away from adults for at least 11-14 days.
- Away from infants, children younger than 16, or pregnant women for at least three to four weeks.

During the daytime, how long should I stay away from infants, children younger than 16, or pregnant women?

I usually recommend at least a week.

What else can I do to minimize contamination?

For the first week, it is recommended to:

- Not prepare food for other people.
- Not share utensils with other people
- Not share towels with other people
- Wash hands very well after using the bathroom
- For men, sit down to urinate
- Wash your towels, bed linens, underwear, and any clothing stained with urine or sweat separately
- Make arrangements for others to provide childcare for infants and very young children

Is there anything I can do to minimize radiation to myself?

- Discuss with your doctor about avoiding excessive doses.
- Fast before the treatment but you need to drink water to keep yourself well hydrated. Fasting makes the radioactive iodine be absorbed faster and get through your gastrointestinal system faster.
- Do not eat immediately after taking the radioactive iodine. Wait at least an hour afterwards.
- Drink plenty of water and urinate frequently.
- If you are being treated for thyroid cancer and have been taken off thyroid medication to increase your TSH, you should not drink water excessively because it

might cause severe low sodium which can be life-threatening. You still need to keep yourself well hydrated. This can be tricky. For most people especially a younger person, you should be okay. For the elderly and especially if you are taking some diuretics, you should not drink too much water.

- Try some sour lozenges to increase production of saliva to reduce the radiation to your salivary glands.
- If you are treated for thyroid cancer, you can resume your thyroid medication the next day.

Chapter 9

Thyroid Hormone Replacement

What is the rate of complication of hypothyroidism (low thyroid) for thyroid nodule treatment?

- Total thyroidectomy-100%
- Lobectomy 20-50%
- Radioactive iodine-50%

The thyroid hormone is very important for your body to function properly, therefore the thyroid hormone needs to be replaced.

What medications on the market can we choose from?

Currently we have the following medications from which you can choose to replace your thyroid hormone:

- Generic levothyroxine (T4)
- Levothroid (T4)
- Levoxyl (T4)
- Synthroid (T4)
- Unithyroid (T4)
- Tirosint (T4)
- Armour thyroid (T4+T3)

- Nature-throid(T4+T3)
- NP thyroid(T4+T3)
- WP-thyroid
- Cytomel (T3)

Which is best?

The most appropriate for you is the best.

What are the most commonly used medications in your clinic?

The most common one I use is generic levothyroxine. I also have a sizable number of patients on the brand name Synthroid and Levoxyl (which has been temporarily discontinued). Some patients are on Armour thyroid, Nature-throid, and NP thyroid. Only a few patients are on Tirosint and cytomel.

Is brand name Synthroid (other brand names in other areas) better than generic?

Theoretically, brand name Synthroid is better. It is more stable since it is manufactured by one manufacturer. Generic levothyroxine is manufactured by many different manufacturers. Even if you get it from the same pharmacy, it may be coming from different manufacturers.

However, for most people the variations introduced are not because of the different manufacturers, it is because they take their medication at different times and may even forget to take it. The most important thing is to take thyroid medication consistently.

If your insurance pays for it or other brand names, I do not have a problem starting patients on Synthroid.

Can I take other brand names instead of Synthroid?

I do not have any problems for my patients to start on any brand if their insurance pays for the other brand names. I have a few patients on Levoxyl but it has temporarily been discontinued. Synthroid is always present in my area of the country.

Can I have an allergy to thyroid medication?

You should not be allergic to thyroid hormone itself but to the "fillers" of the pill.

What "fillers" are present in Synthroid pill?

Acacia, confectioner's sugar (contains corn starch), lactose monohydrate, magnesium stearate, povidone, and talc. Different doses of medication also contain different coloring materials.

What is acacia? Could I be allergic to it?

Acacia is used to make the shape of the pill. It comes from shrubs and woods. Some people are allergic to it. If you have an allergy to tree pollens you might have an allergy to acacia too.

Shunzhong Shawn Bao, MD

I am lactose intolerant, and I saw Synthroid has lactose in it. Can I still take it?

The dose of lactose in the pill is very, very low. You should not have a problem taking it.

What is povidone? Is it toxic?

Povidone is a polymerized form of vinylpyrolidone, which is a white hygroscopic powder that is easily soluble in water and used as a dispersing and suspending agent in drugs like Synthroid.

It seems safe and I have not seen any research about allergies to povidone. People can have a mild or severe allergy to povidone-iodine which is used as skin disinfectant.

What is talc? Is it cancer causing?

Talc is a naturally occurring mineral mined from the earth that is composed of magnesium, silicon, oxygen, and hydrogen. Chemically, talc is a hydrous magnesium silicate with a chemical formula of $Mg_3Si_4O_{10}(OH)_2$.
Talc has many uses in cosmetics and other personal care products; in food such as rice and chewing gum; and in the manufacturing of tablets.
The cousin of talc-asbestos is a cancer causing agent. There is no evidence to show that talc causes cancer or allergies.

Synthroid comes in different colors. What are the color agents in the pill?

Synthroid has 12 different strengths (mcg) with 12 different colors.

Table. Synthroid tablet color and additives.

Strength (mcg)	Color additive(s)
25	orange--FD&C Yellow No. 6 Aluminum Lake
50	white------None
75	violet----FD&C Red No. 40 Aluminum Lake, and FD&C Blue No. 2 Aluminum Lake
88	olive------FD&C Blue No. 1 Aluminum Lake, FD&C Yellow No. 6 Aluminum Lake, D&C Yellow No. 10 Aluminum Lake
100	yellow---D&C Yellow No. 10 Aluminum Lake, FD&C Yellow No. 6 Aluminum Lake
112	rose--D&C Red No. 27 & 30 Aluminum Lake
125	brown-FD&C Yellow No. 6 Aluminum Lake, FD&C Red No. 40 Aluminum Lake, FD&C Blue No. 1 Aluminum Lake

Table (continued). Synthroid tablet color and its additives.

Strength (mcg)	Color additive(s)
137	Turquoise-FD&C Blue No. 1 Aluminum Lake
150	blue-FD&C Blue No. 2 Aluminum Lake
175	lilac-FD&C Blue No. 1 Aluminum Lake, D&C Red No. 27 & 30 Aluminum Lake
200	pink-FD&C Red No. 40 Aluminum Lake
300	green-D&C Yellow No. 10 Aluminum Lake, FD&C Yellow No. 6 Aluminum Lake, FD&C Blue No. 1 Aluminum Lake

Is aluminum lake toxic?

Aluminum lake is aluminum oxide. It is believed to be nontoxic.

Can I have an allergy to dyes?

Yes, it is possible. If suspected, you can try the dosage of 50 ug which does not have coloring agents. I used this as a base to make different doses. The following is my scheme to make different doses.

- 25 ug: ½ tab daily
- 50 ug: 1 tab daily
- 75 ug: 1 and ½ tabs daily
- 88 ug: 5 days of 2 tabs daily, and 2 days of 1 tab daily
- 100 ug: 2 tabs daily
- 112 ug: 6 days of 2 tabs daily and one day of 3.5 tabs.
- 125 ug: 2.5 tabs daily
- 137 ug:3 tabs daily for 6 daily and 1 tab for one day.
- 150 ug: 3 tabs daily
- 175 ug:3.5 tabs daily
- 200 ug: 4 tabs daily
- 250 ug: 5 tabs daily
- 300 ug: 6 tabs daily

What is the color scheme for other T4 brands?

Most of them use the same color scheme, but there are some differences.

Strength (ug)	Levothroid (Actavis)	Levoxyl (Pfizer)	Synthroid (Abbvie)	Unithroid (Watson)
25	orange	orange	orange	peach
50	white	white	white	white
75	violet	purple	violet	purple
88	mint green	olive	olive	olive
100	yellow	yellow	yellow	yellow
112	rose	rose	rose	rose
125	brown	brown	brown	tan
137	deep blue	dark blue	turquoise	Not available
150	blue	blue	blue	blue
175	lilac	turquoise	lilac	lilac
200	pink	pink	pink	pink
300	green	green	green	green

Is the gel form-Tirosint better?

It is believed that the gel form Tirosint has better absorption. Patients with atrophic gastritis, patients taking anti-acid medications, or patients with a history of gastric bypass surgery could benefit from this due to absorption issues. I do not worry about this too much, I usually just increase the dose. The gel form is more expensive. If your insurance will pay for it and you believe it works better for you, I do not have a problem prescribing it.

I have patients who have malabsorption and I have prescribed 500-1000 ug of levothyroxine. I wanted to try Tirosint but was not able to get insurance to pay for it.

What fillers does Tirosint have?

Inactive ingredients: gelatin, glycerin, and water.
People might have an allergic reaction to gelatin, but usually not to glycerin.

Does Tirosint have color coding?

No, Tirosint does not have color coding on the gel. If you are allergic to color agents, this version might be a good option for you. However, if your insurance doesn't pay for it or it is too expensive for you, you can use my scheme to form different dose with colorless 50 ug pills.

Shunzhong Shawn Bao, MD

On the boxes, the color coding is as follows.

Strength (ug)	Color on the box
13	green
25	peach
50	white
100	purple
112	yellow
125	brown
150	blue

Does Tirosint cause less allergic reactions?

Yes. Tirosint has fewer fillers and no coloring agents added. If you are looking for "pure" thyroid hormone replacement. This is the purest.

I have patients who also claimed to have an allergic reaction to it. Presumably they are allergic to gelatin. Many vaccines also have gelatin. If you are allergic to vaccines then you might be allergic to Tirosint. but vaccines have more allergens in them.

How are Tirosint capsules supplied?

They are supplied as follows: Boxes of 56 capsules, consisting of 8 blisters with 7 capsules each.

What is the best time to take T4 formulations like generic levothyroxine, Synthroid, Levoxyl, Levothroid, Unithroid, or Tirosint?

It is recommended to take them early in the morning on an empty stomach. Ideally take it 60 minutes before you drink anything except water, eat, or take any other medications.

However, most of my patients are not able to do that. I usually ask my patients to put the medication and a cup of water on their nightstand the night before and, as soon as they open their eyes, pop in the medication with a cup of water. During the night, you lose a lot of water so it is good for you to drink a cup of water when you wake up.

Can I take T4 formulations like generic levothyroxine, Synthroid, Levoxyl, Levothroid, Unithroid, or Tirosint at night?

I have patients who cannot take it early in the morning, so I ask them to take it before going to bed. I urge them to not eat any snacks after dinner. Bedtime and dinner should be at least four hours apart.

What should I do if I forget a day?

It is best not to forget, but life happens, so if you forget, I recommend you double it the next day.

Shunzhong Shawn Bao, MD

Do you have any options for my son who is 16 years old? He never remembers to take his meds and I cannot be after him every day to take them.

Your son is not alone. Lots of teens are not good at taking medications. They either forget, do not want to take it, or wake up too late. It is very challenging for teens to take thyroid medication.

I recommend my patients to choose one day each week and to take seven pills all at once. It is not ideal but at least you know they consistently get taken.

I have malabsorption. What options do I have?

Tirosint may be better for you if your insurance will pay for it. Otherwise, I would just increase your dose.

However, I have patients who have such severe malabsorption that we must give intravenous levothyroxine periodically and insurance usually will balk at paying for it.

I have Crohn's disease. Do you have any recommendations for me?

Crohn's disease is an inflammatory bowel disease. It can be very challenging with flair ups and changes in absorption rates in the body. You can try Tirosint which has a better absorption rate. The key issue is to check your thyroid function more often.

I am also taking iron and calcium supplements. Any extra precautions?

Iron and calcium affect thyroid medication absorption significantly. I recommend you take your calcium or iron pills at least four hours after taking your thyroid medication. If you take your thyroid medication in the morning, then I recommend you take iron or calcium at supper or at night.

I am also taking an osteoporosis medication called bisphosphonates-like Actonel (risedronate), Fosamax (alendronate), Boniva (ibandronate), Pamidronate. Can I take my thyroid hormone with these medications?

These medications also require you to take them early in the morning on an empty stomach and then wait 60 minutes before you eat or drink anything else except water.

Since these medications are usually taken once a week or once a month, I am not particularly worried about these.

If you take your thyroid medication and osteoporosis medication together with your osteoporosis meds, it might affect thyroid medication absorption. Since T4 formulations (generic levothyroxine, Synthroid, Levoxyl, Levothroid, Unithroid, or Tirosint) come with half-life of seven days, one day of lower absorption will not affect your blood thyroid level too much. Your thyroid hormone level will be stable.

If you do not want to take them together, you can also omit your thyroid hormone on the day you are taking the bisphosphonates and then double up your thyroid medication the next day.

However, if you are newly starting your bisphosphonates, I recommend having your thyroid function checked in six weeks and adjusting your dose as needed.

I am also taking acid reflux / stomach medications - H pump inhibitors - -like Nexium (esoprazole), Omeprazole, Pantoprazole, Lansoprazole, Dexilant (dexlansoprazole), or Aciphex (rabeprazole) medications. My doctors tell me to take them on an empty stomach. What should I do?

These medications will reduce thyroid medication absorption. The good news is that your doctor can always increase the thyroid medication dose as needed. I first let my patients take their thyroid medication with these medications together empty stomach to see if we can get their thyroid level stable.

Another option is to take the thyroid medication at night. However, these patients are also taking other medications at night which might affect their thyroid medication absorption. It is better to take them together in the morning.

I have patients who like to take thyroid medication 30 minutes before taking these mentioned medications. This option is also acceptable. The key issue is consistency.

Certainly if you start later you will need to check your thyroid function in 4-6 weeks after you are started on H pump inhibitors to make sure you are taking sufficient thyroid medication.

I am taking antacids, what should I pay attention to?

If you are taking antacids like aluminum hydroxide, magnesium hydroxide, Alka-seltzer, Pepto, Maalox, Mylanta(aluminum hydroxide/magnesium hydroxide), Rolaids, or Tums; these medications should be taken at least four hours after thyroid medication. I strongly recommend you take your thyroid medication early in the morning on an empty stomach with a cup of room temperature or warm water.

If you are taking your antacids periodically, you really need to take your thyroid medication first, take it consistently early in the morning on an empty stomach, and wait 45-60 minutes before you eat, drink, or take anything else. These antacids should not be taken within four hours of thyroid medications.

I am taking carafate for my stomach ulcer. I heard this medication can affect thyroid medication absorption. What should I do?

It is true that carafate reduces thyroid medication absorption. This medication might be taken 4 times a day and needs to be taken 1 hour before a meal. In this situation, I recommend taking your thyroid medication 30 minutes before taking carafate with a cup of warm water. Close monitoring and adjusting thyroid medication is strongly recommended.

What other medications should I pay attention to while taking thyroid medication?

If you are taking any of the following medications, you should take them at least four hours apart from thyroid medication. Consistency is the key. Let your thyroid doctor know so the dose can be adjusted:

- Cholestyramine-cholesterol medication.
- Colesevelam--cholesterol medication.
- Selevemer-lower phosphorus in renal failure patients.
- Raloxifene (Evista)-breast cancer prevention and treating osteoporosis.

There are certainly many other medications which might affect thyroid medication absorption. Keep taking the medications four hours apart if you can.

I was told that I cannot take my thyroid medication with coffee. However, I always rush in the morning. There is no way that I can wait 60 minutes before I drink my coffee. Are you sure I absolutely cannot drink coffee?

Life is complicated as you described and taking thyroid medication certainly makes it more complicated. I am very liberal: If you are willing to promise that you drink the same coffee and same time every day, I will let you try. We can always adjust your thyroid medication dose.

Another option is to take your thyroid medication at night. After dinner you are not supposed to eat snacks for at least 4 hours.

I cannot wait 60 minutes before I eat my breakfast. What should I do?

Milk and soy products, coffee and other fibers all affect thyroid medication absorption. As I recommended before, prepare yourself a cup of water on your nightstand the night before. As soon as you open your eyes, you can pop in your thyroid medication. After you get washed and dressed , 30 minutes might have passed. This is not 60 minutes as recommended, but it will be acceptable.

I also have patients taking their thyroid medication when they wake up in the middle of night or early morning. You are allowed to take at that time.

Whatever you do, if you can do it consistently it is not a big deal. We can always adjust your dose.

How do you decide which dose to start?

I use the information of the patient's weight, lean body mass, pregnancy status, cause of hypothyroidism (RAI or surgery), degree of TSH elevation, age, history of cardiovascular disease, and other conditions including the presence of cardiac disease. The most important thing is to have follow up and adjust your medication. It is very important to start right, but more important is to adjust and take your medication correctly and consistently.

Shunzhong Shawn Bao, MD

I swear that I feel better when I am on Armour thyroid. My former endocrinologist did not believe me. Do you believe me?

I believe you, and I have 20% of my patients who like to take a desiccated thyroid product like Armour thyroid.

The thyroid gland is complicated. The thyroid gland secretes a variety of iodinated and non-iodinated molecules that collectively play important roles during our prenatal and adult lives. We do not understand them yet. When I was an Endocrine Fellow at Washington University School of Medicine, I had a fellow classmate who did research on calcitonin. He claimed that replacement of calcitonin affects feelings of wellbeing.

My approach to this request is to keep an open mind. I acknowledged that a T4 formulation like levothyroxine is the mainstream supplement and it is very easy to take. Most patients are doing very well on this. I let patients try other formulations if they are not happy about their current medication. I do let patients know that there are many reasons which might cause them to not feel well that we cannot fix on thyroid medications. I also let my patients know that sometimes we will have to use desiccated thyroid 2 times a day due to high levels of T3 in it. The dose difference between each batch may be larger even from the same manufacturer, and sometimes it is very difficult to have a right dose. Also the T4, T3 and other molecules might also vary from batch to batch. Dessicated thyroid also has a lab test that is sometimes difficult for a non-specialist to interpret.

The manufacturer also advises that a potential risk of product contamination with porcine and bovine viral or other adventitious agents cannot be ruled out.

What is Armour thyroid anyway?

Armour Thyroid for oral use is a natural preparation derived from porcine thyroid glands. They provide 38 mcg levothyroxine (T4) and 9 mcg liothyronine (T3) per grain of thyroid (equivalent of 60 mg).

What is WP thyroid or Nature-throid?

They are two other products from desiccated pig thyroid. I treat them the same as Armour thyroid, however the dose forms are slightly different.

What is the dose equivalent between desiccated thyroid and T4 preparations like levothyroxine?

Usually, I start 100 ug of levothyroxine converted to 60 mg (grain) of Armour thyroid or 65 mg (grain) of WP thyroid or Nature-throid.

The Armour thyroid and NP thyroid has a dose increment of 15 mg (equivalent to levothyroxine 25 ug).

The WP thyroid and Nature-throid have dose increments of 16.25 mg equivalent to levothyroxine 25 ug..

Table of the dose conversions between commonly used thyroid replacement preparation.

Levothyroxine Mcg	Armour grain(mg)	WP thyroid grain(mg)	Nature-throid grain(mg)
25	¼(15)	¼(16.25)	¼(16.25)
50	½(30)	½(32.5)	½(32.5)
75		¾(48.75)	¾(48.75)
88			
100	1(60)	1(65)	1(65)
112			
125		1.25(81.25)	1/25(81.25)
137			
150	1.5(90)	1.5(97.5)	1.5(97.5)
175		1.75(113.75)	1.75(113.75)
200	2(120)	2(130)	2(130)
			2.25(146.25)
			2.5(162.5)
300	3(180)		3(195)
	4(240)		4(260)
	5(300)		5(325)

What are the inactive ingredients in the pill?

The inactive ingredients are calcium stearate, dextrose, microcrystalline cellulose, sodium starch glycolate, and opadry white.

Can I have an allergy to natural desiccated thyroid?

Yes, you can.

Can I take my Armour thyroid or other desiccated thyroid at night?

Theoretically it is okay to take it at night. The thyroid effect in cells needs a few hours to work. However, I still have patients complaining about it affecting their sleep. My point is that you can try it and if it does not affect your sleep, you can take it at bedtime.

I am on a thyroid supplement. Do I need to take extra iodine?

No, you do not. You already are being supplemented with iodine product of the thyroid hormone.

I am on a thyroid supplement. Do I need to take a selenium supplement?

Selenium helps you to convert T4 to the active hormone T3. However, most people do not have a selenium deficiency and you might not need to take it. If you want to take it, it is acceptable and it might help you. However, if you take too much, it can cause toxicity.

My TSH is low. Why did my doctor reduce my thyroid medication?

As we discussed previously, TSH is like a thermostat. If your thyroid hormone level is too high, then TSH is going to be reduced. The opposite is true also. If your thermostat ramps up it means the temperature at your house is too low. If the TSH is too high it means your thyroid hormone level is too low. That is why when you TSH is low your doctor will lower your thyroid medication; if your TSH is too high, your doctor will increase your medication.

Just remember, the TSH level is always opposite to your thyroid hormone level. The premise is that you have a normal pituitary gland.

I heard that taking thyroid medication can help me to lose weight. Can I take more?

It is really a bad idea to take more thyroid medication to lose weight. Too much thyroid medication may cause atrial fibrillation which will increase your risk for stroke. Too much thyroid medication can also cause osteoporosis. These are the two most serious side effects.

Chapter 10

Questions About Thyroid Cancer Screening, Benign Nodule and Thyroid Cancer Follow-up

Should I have a thyroid cancer screening?

It is not recommended for the general population to have thyroid cancer screening.

However if you have one of the following situations, I recommend you have a thyroid cancer screening. Depending on the findings you and your doctor will decide the screening frequency.

- Significant family history of thyroid cancer
- Family history of medullary thyroid cancer
- Family history of MEN II (multiple endocrine neoplasia)
- Family history of Cowden syndrome
- Family history of APC (adenomatous polyposis)
- Family history of Gardner syndrome

I have some small nodules (<1 cm). How often should I have thyroid ultrasound?

We all want to do less. This is a good thing in this situation.

Here are my recommendations:

- Nodule < 1 cm and without high risk ultrasound features (irregular border, undefined border, lobulated margin, very hypoechoic, calcification (microcalcification, broken egg shell calcification), taller than width), you can recheck every two to five years.
- If you have nodules with the above features, I recommend you have an ultrasound at least once a year. If there are multiple risk features, you might discuss with your doctor to proceed with thyroid nodule FNA.

How often should I follow my benign thyroid nodules?

Even if your nodule proved to be benign by FNA, you still need to have a follow up. I usually follow up benign nodules once a year. Benign nodules also tend to grow but if it grows too fast, then I recommend repeating a FNA. If the nodule has multiple ultrasound risk features, even FNA benign nodules, I still recommend surgery or more close follow-up.

I was diagnosed with thyroid cancer. What is my chance of dying from thyroid cancer?

It is estimated that in 2016, there were 64,300 new cases diagnosed and total of 630,000 patients were living with thyroid cancer in United States. A total of 1980 patients died of thyroid cancer.

If you have a differentiated thyroid cancer <1 cm, the chance of dying from thyroid cancer is close to zero.

If you are 45 years old or younger and have differentiated thyroid cancer and content in the thyroid, your 10 year survival is 100%.

Even if you have more advanced cancer, you still will live long and well with thyroid cancer, although the prognosis is not as good as less advanced cancer.

I have thyroid cancer. Can I avoid surgery?

So far, I do not have any patients who were found to have thyroid cancer and did not want to have surgery. Before doing the FNA procedure, I let my patients know the possible results and accordingly what we are expect to do. If the patient does not want to have surgery for some reason, I may not proceed with the FNA.

I have had thyroid surgery and was found to have thyroid cancer. Do I have to have a radioactive iodine treatment?

No, not everybody with thyroid cancer needs radioactive iodine treatment (ablation). You and your doctor will discuss the necessity of a radioactive adjuvant treatment.

If we decide to have the radioactive treatment, how long do I have to be off thyroid medication replacement?

If your doctor and you decide to have thyroid medication withdrawn, you will usually be off thyroid medication for three to four weeks. Your doctor will check your TSH to make sure it is above 35. Thyroid medication withdrawal can have some complications like significant fatigue, weight gain, constipation, and depression. Other complications like feeling cold or hair loss can also occur.

If it has been over 4 weeks, and your TSH is still less than 35, usually something is wrong. I would stop the process and urge your insurance company to pay for Thyrogen (recombinant TSH) to finish the iodine ablation.

Is there any way I can avoid thyroid medication withdrawal?

Yes, we have recombinant human TSH injection (Thyrogen) to give you. If your insurance will pay for it, I recommend everybody use it. During those three to four week thyroid hormone withdrawals, the complications are not good.

Before radioactive iodine treatment, how long do I have to be on a low iodine diet?

I recommend at least two weeks. For a low-iodine diet (stay away from high-iodine food, please see Chapter 1 and Chapter 8).

How often should I get a whole body iodine scan?

I usually only recommend one time after the radioactive iodine treatment. If the initial scan was negative, I do not follow up with more scans unless your cancer marker goes up.

Do I still need a thyroid ultrasound since I have had my thyroid removed already?

Yes, thyroid ultrasounds are a good tool to monitor thyroid cancer recurrence. You should have a thyroid ultrasound periodically.

How often should I have my cancer marker thyroglobulin checked?

It depends, but I check my patients at least once a year. Under some circumstances, I might check every three months.

Do I need to have a CT/MRI/PET scan for my thyroid cancer follow up?

For most patients, you do not need those tests.

Do I need to see an oncologist for my thyroid cancer?

If you need to see an oncologist, your endocrinologist will refer you to one. Otherwise, your endocrinologist will be the main person taking care of your thyroid cancer treatment following surgery with or without iodine treatment.

Do I need chemotherapy?

For most patients, you will not need chemotherapy therefore you will not need to see an oncologist.

Do I need radiation therapy?

Most patients will not need radiation therapy. You might need iodine ablation which is different from radiation therapy.

Printed in Great Britain
by Amazon

19723692R00068